ALONE WITH DEMENTIA

by

Margaret Jeremiah

William Sessions Limited
York, England

ISBN 1 85072 304 4

For Keith

Thanks to
Fleur Bradnock
who did the typing, sorted me out and without
whom I could not have managed.

Printed in 11 point Plantin Typeface
from Author's Disk
by Sessions of York
The Ebor Press
York, England

Contents

Foreword

Perhaps more than many diseases, the dementias are a family affair. When we ask patients and carers in our day care facilities about what they hope for from our services, sharing the burden of care and sharing expert knowledge with carers emerge as important issues. The different causes of dementia, from a biological point of view, and the psychological and social overlay that make dementia more of a burden than it needs to be, mean that diagnosis and referral to specialist services is often delayed. Too often people are denied access to that help until late in the disease. The arrival of medication for Alzheimer's disease is resulting in more people being referred early to the specialist services and this may help avoid these services being seen as a "last resort". However, the UK is the only member of the Organisation for Economic Cooperation and Development whose proportion of healthcare spending on the over 65s is currently reducing, so services are likely to continue to be stretched!

The area of spirituality and dementia is currently enjoying a great deal of interest. The Christian Council on Ageing has a Dementia Group that has been working for ten years to raise awareness of the spiritual needs of people with dementia. It has taken a broad approach, recognising that people express and satisfy spiritual needs in different ways. For some people, formal religion is the key. Others take a more humanistic approach, concentrating on the importance of interpersonal relationships as mediators of meaning. Quakers testify to "that of God in everyone" and in some ways bridge the gap between more formal religious expression and those who would do without God altogether.

The account you will read here comes from a Quaker perspective. It is a moving personal account, from the perspective of a loving partner taking on the role of "carer", of the unfolding of a dementing illness, complicated by poor sight. It shows many of the triumphs and failures of current services. If you are reading this as a family member or friend of someone with dementia, it may help you feel less alone. If you are reading it as a professional provider of services, I hope it will move you to redouble efforts to provide services that are sensitive to the human needs of both people with dementia and their families and friends. If you are reading it as a commissioner of services or as somebody with political "clout", I hope you will consider how you can ensure fair priority to improving services for people with dementia and their families.

John Wattis
Professor of Psychiatry for Older People
University of Huddersfield   January 2003

Introduction

All of us either die young or grow old - that is inevitable - but it is not inevitable that, as Shakespeare put it, we all become 'sans everything'. Even when we live to be over 90, and more of us are living to 100 now, half of us will retain all our faculties until the end. It is no longer believed that senile dementia creeps up on everyone slowly but inevitably as we get older, but although much work has been done in some cities and universities, old fears and beliefs about old age and dementia still remain among a surprising number of otherwise well-informed people. Many such people choose to retire to unspoilt countryside, which has many advantages, but there are also disadvantages as they get older. What these will be is difficult to forecast.

This book is about one person's experience in a village of fewer than 600 people on the electoral roll. Everyone's experience will of course be different but if we can break through the barrier of fear and horror that many people – including doctors – have of mental breakdown, it will be a step in the right direction. I have just been reading Margaret Drabble's critique of William Wordsworth's *Idiot Boy*. She points out that Wordsworth does not deny that disgust and aversion are possible reactions but he says quite bluntly and firmly that they are not a moral attitude. To clarify to myself why humans should be treated as human even when their brains have ceased to function properly, I turned to the religious philosopher/palaeontologist, Pierre Teilhard de Chardin, and found in the Introduction to his *The Phenomenon of Man* the famous English scientist Sir Julian Huxley saying 'The brain alone is not responsible for the mind, even though it is a necessary organ for its manifestation.'

This was very important for me as a person who had 'bonded' with someone for nearly 60 years but was now not recognised and could no longer share memories or experiences.

I had had no medical or psychological training and at the age of 80 years I had to care for someone of similar age with this mysterious and (at the moment) incurable disease. This is not a new disease but mostly affects older people and as the population is living to a greater average age so the disadvantages of old old age are becoming more common and there are not enough trained and experienced people to go round. If there are two of you and you live in a sparsely populated rural area you have to cope as best you can on your own.

In 1981, soon after we moved here from Hampshire, there was a man in the village, James B., who suffered from dementia. This was the only other case I heard of in the village. I appreciate the value of confidentiality but there are sometimes cases where help would be more readily available if this rule were not so rigidly adhered to. Jim and his wife Gladys were younger than we were. He had been a teacher of physics and a very clever man. They often passed our house as Jim had a passion for walking but as he could never say where he had been his wife followed close behind him to make sure he came to no harm. If I had known more then I might have been more able to help them. I did ask them in for a rest and refreshment but although Gladys was glad to be invited she felt she had to refuse as she knew her husband would not come in and would not like to wait for her. Jim eventually died at home and his widow and I became good friends and went together to well organised talks about bereavement. With the help of organisations such as the Hospice movement, Cruse and other organisations that provide counselling, the traumas that people experience are better understood, but there is still a long way to go before there is enough help for the lone, often elderly, partner of anyone with dementia. Incidentally, Gladys told me that when she wanted to prepare a meal she had to persuade Jim to practise his flute so she could hear where he was but get on with her cooking in peace. I could not do this with my husband as although he enjoyed listening to music he had never learned to play an instrument. He did have some lessons on the classical guitar when he retired but the advent of dementia made this too difficult. Gladys soon left the village and went to Bedford to be with her children. She died there a few years later.

It is more comfortable to assume that people with dementia have no knowledge of what is happening to them and no awareness of who or where they are and the best thing to do is to shut them away and forget them. Unfortunately this is not usually true, as most people who have known the patient well have always suspected. One woman kept a diary for ten years and after her death her daughter wrote to the Alzheimer's Society and told how her mother had never been informed that she was suffering from dementia, though she had known all along that something terrible was happening to her brain. Just imagine the lonely terror of that poor woman. There was also a story in *The Friend* (the weekly newsletter of The Quakers) about an elderly German man who could not speak and appeared to understand nothing and was treated by his grandsons as a non-person. Suddenly he heard a grandson trying to do his English language homework. The grandfather seemed to recognise the language he had learned as a child and was then able to converse with an English-speaking friend.

Some research has been done (and published by the Joseph Rowntree Foundation) by Kate Allan of the University of Stirling to follow on from work also at Stirling by Malcolm Goldsmith called *Hearing the Voice of People with Dementia*. Kate Allan dealt entirely with professional carers in institutions, the idea being to find out what people with dementia thought about the way they were treated. In most public health situations now patients are expected to make choices, though until recently people with dementia were not thought able to express an opinion, being more like animated corpses than real people. Kate Allan found the staff very willing to co-operate with her research and they found that the effort to communicate with their charges made their work more rewarding. It is interesting to note that Kate Allan is well aware of the risk of over identification, burn-out and stress and if this is the case in a professional setting, how much more is this true when two people have 'bonded' for many years in a home situation where communication is taken for granted.

CHAPTER 1

Situations and people change with the passing of time

When Keith (my husband) and I first came to live in this village, twenty years ago, we did not feel isolated. We had our boat in the dyke round the corner, two bicycles and a car in the garage, and two pairs of strong legs that could and often did carry us for several miles without complaint. Norwich was only twelve miles in one direction and Great Yarmouth about the same distance in the other. We enjoyed doing whatever was needed in the house and garden and often had friends and families to stay. We had a very jolly party to celebrate our Golden Wedding in 1991 but after that things began to go wrong. Keith had two minor accidents with the car and in 1993 he was registered blind with a burst blood-vessel in the macular of his only good eye.

We joined the Macular Degeneration Society as soon as Keith was registered blind and they immediately sent him an invaluable tape, by an eminent specialist, which described the cause and effect of the disease. On the other side of the tape a youngish social worker told how he coped with this handicap in his work. Keith, with the encouragement of the Macular Degeneration Society, made copies of the tape and distributed them to local doctors. Our own doctor (who has since retired) was very appreciative and said that before he heard the tape he was not aware of some of the symptoms that Keith had described and which were mentioned on the tape. The local association for the blind was also very helpful and sent a pleasant young woman who helped us fill in the difficult form for Attendance Allowance and arranged for us to have a Talking Book machine delivered. The Association for the Blind also had a good display of aids for the blind and partially sighted people and a nursing home and some sheltered flats. I was already finding it difficult

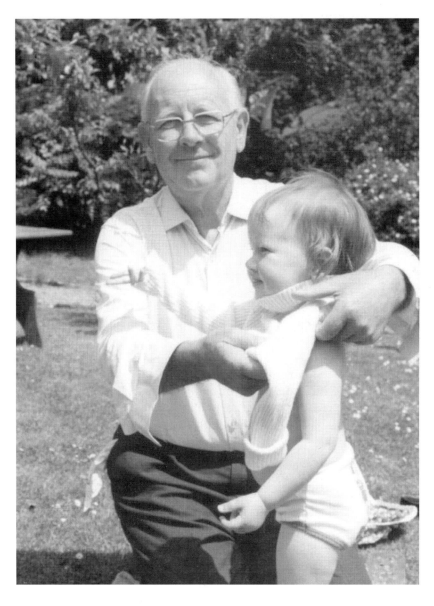

He loved children.

to give Keith all the help and attention he needed together with all the paperwork involved with looking after the house, car, garden, finance, licensing, repairing and redecorating and so on, but the flats were not available for couples. I tried various other establishments but the only place that offered us accommodation together was very small and far from any friends and relations.

The jobs we had enjoyed doing together became too much for me and the effort to cope with the work for which he had always taken responsibility before had to be learned, which is not easy at an age when one would be glad of a little Tender Loving Care oneself and when one is caring for someone with a very strange illness, while appearing as fit as ever. I had worked, before I was married, on the administrative side of a hospital and for three years before the children were born I was in charge of a hostel for aged and infirm evacuees, but although Keith had always had difficulty with swallowing and had nearly died of blood poisoning in 1987, I had always managed to look after him until he developed these mental problems, and of course I was older. At one time there would have been servants or unmarried children to share the burden but now even most of our friends and relations had died or were too old and far away to be any help. Our youngest daughter did her best but, although she lives only three miles away, she has four children and two jobs and a husband who is often away so she could not spare the time for us.

Keith had to give up driving of course, but fortunately I could drive. At first I would put him on a train for Norwich (the station was three miles away) and with his white stick and local knowledge he managed very well, going from one optician to another trying to find something that would enable him to use the hitherto 'lazy eye'. This gave me some time for respite or to get things done. I soon found, however, that he caught the next train back and wandered about the station until I met him at the prearranged time. He had by then a talking watch, again thanks to the Association for the Blind.

When he went to see the doctor Keith asked him if he had Alzheimer's. To which the doctor seems to have replied 'If you had you would not be asking that question'. I do not think the doctor realised, and I certainly did not, that he had suffered a series of minor strokes, probably caused by the high blood pressure that had troubled him, defeating all medication, since the age of forty. This, according to the book obtained from the Alzheimer's Society by one of our daughters, can cause what the experts call multi-infarct dementia. Dementia was not mentioned at the time and I put any strangeness in his behaviour down to his blindness. As John Bailey says in his book about his wife (Iris Murdoch) when she descended into dementia: 'The disease (in her case Alzheimer's) creeps up unnoticed by the nearest and dearest but possibly sub-consciously suspected by both the carer and the partner, but in the folk tradition of senility inevitably coming on gradually with age, provided a protective shield behind which all our society has crouched for too long.'

Keith was very fond of plays and classical music, so I took him to everything he said he would like that was on in Norwich, but before long I noticed his attention span had become so short that we had hardly found our seats before he wanted to go home again.

One advantage of living in a small village where there is little public transport, or traffic of any sort, is that Keith could not go far by himself or come to much harm. There is a lot of water about but he seemed to know that it could be dangerous and kept well away from it. He used sometimes to go to the Post Office to get our pensions, and on Fridays to the Pub, to get our fish and chips. Sometimes he got lost and was brought home by strangers. He also delivered the Parish Magazine but I soon decided to take him in the car and stop outside the appropriate houses. To my horror I found he would sometimes deliver several at one house and nothing at another. When I remonstrated his reply was that he was required to deliver a certain number and that was what he had done.

Keith had been very choosy about getting a solicitor to supervise and update our wills since the solicitor (who was also a friend) we had in Hampshire died. Fortunately we had recently agreed on a friend who lived at Wells-next-the-Sea. He strongly advised that I should have Power of Attorney. Keith seemed quite happy about that idea and so it was agreed, although I did not like what it appeared to suggest. Later this went to the Court of Protection and all the children had to be officially notified - altogether a necessary but expensive business.

CHAPTER 2

Blindness was bad enough but that was not all

Keith was very restless and was always asking where we were going for a holiday this year. One year I took him to Harare to visit our eldest daughter who was there with her husband, who works with the European Union in Africa. Keith seemed happy to be there, but I picked up a bug on the plane and was ill most of the time. However it was lovely to be looked after. Another year I arranged a coach tour of the Rocky Mountains and a trip up the coast of Alaska in a cruise ship, with Saga. We enjoyed seeing a niece and her family in Vancouver but even Saga, that claims to specialise in caring for old people, seemed to find it difficult to provide for the blind and some of our fellow travellers were distinctly unhelpful. My final effort was to take Keith to a self-catering flat. This was in Cornwall, where we had spent our honeymoon and where Keith had many happy childhood memories. We were glad to visit many friends and relations we had known well in the past, but this time I had all the work and driving to do.

When we were at home I took Keith to our usual Quaker Meeting for Worship, where he behaved perfectly but on the way back he always said 'That was a waste of time wasn't it?' I also took him to a discussion group in Norwich once a month and I got very cross when he embarrassed me by saying 'You have all got cars, why don't you all go home to bed? You are not doing any good here.' He did not seem to be aware of what other people were doing or saying.

I became seriously worried about the state of Keith's mind when we were returning home to Norfolk from Keswick. We had as usual spent a week in a hired static caravan beside Derwent Water with our children and their children, their friends and their children. We had enjoyed watching them in and on the water with their various craft. After the holiday we had to vacate the caravan at 10 am and broke the journey by spending the night at a Travel Lodge. We had hardly started on this occasion when Keith said 'Isn't it about time you turned round and took us home?' to which I replied 'We are going home.' I was a bit flabbergasted when he asked 'Your home or my home?' It transpired that he thought we had been in a house by the sea in Cornwall. I never did find out who he thought I was.

Shortly after we returned home he used the memory button on the telephone and ordered our youngest daughter to return his mother and his wife who he thought she had been keeping from him. His mother died 30 years ago and I (his wife) was sitting beside him. I asked who he thought I was and without hesitation he replied 'A friend we are very fond of.' I followed this with 'Who do you mean by "We"?' His reply was 'My wife, my mother and me of course'. Our daughter-in-law told me that when they were out for a short walk together, Keith had suddenly had one of his rare lucid spells and said it was like coming out of a dream. He knew it was nonsense for a man of his age to be looking for his mother like a little boy. But in the dream he did not doubt it. This is why it seems to me to be cruel to ignore people with dementia however irrational they appear most of the time. At about this time he started to walk into other peoples' houses, usually when I was in the kitchen preparing our evening meal. He always said he was looking for his mother but as she was also 'Mrs Jeremiah' older women just turned him round and sent him home saying 'I'm sure you will find her there'. Some even telephoned me to make sure he got back safely. Others, and who can blame them when a man they hardly knew walked in out of the dark, were afraid and might eventually have called the police and created an unhappy situation. The husbands said they feared the dogs would savage him – another scenario I could not accept with equanimity. I dare not lock the door as he was already showing signs of rage when thwarted. I once objected to being cold when he took all the bedding for himself - he then thumped me. When I told him this as the explanation for my sleeping in another room he said 'I would never do anything like that to you. It must have been one of the other chaps.' This was too much for my sense of humour and I asked 'How many chaps did you think were sleeping in our bed?'

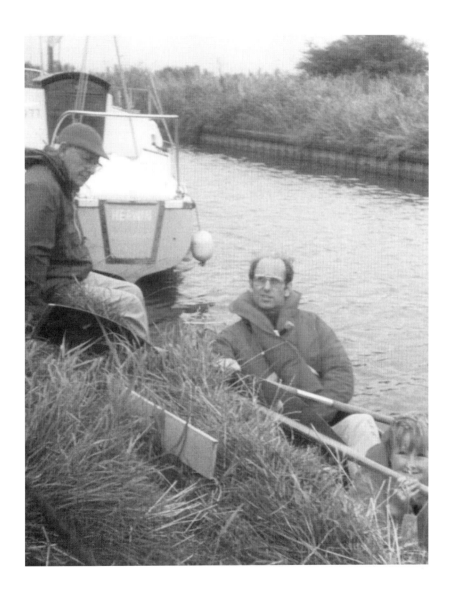

With son and grandson; all called Keith and all fond of water and boats.

A neighbour and her husband sat with Keith once to give me some respite but they could not do it again as they had a sick father to look after. They suggested that, via the doctor, we could get help from the Social Services. We got an appointment with the (new) doctor who asked Keith the usual questions about the name of the Prime Minister etc., which I thought he answered as well as I could have done in the time allowed, but the doctor seemed satisfied and said he would report his findings to Dr Tawse, who was the Mental Health officer for the area, and she would soon call on us.

When Dr Tawse came, Keith refused to answer any of her questions. She asked me if he was very clinging and said that she would need to examine him in her hospital but in the meantime she got the Social Worker to arrange for him to attend a Respite Centre (at Wroxham) once a week. As I told the doctor, Keith would not go anywhere without me or let me go anywhere without him. This meant I had to take him and slip out again before the door was locked. He was furious about this and I knew that I could not get him there many more times. If I had known more I could have stayed with him a few times and he might have got used to it. The place where the Respite Centre was held was a fine house but the main building was used as a Residential Home. The Day (Respite) Centre was in rather cramped accommodation in out-buildings and was run by a kind motherly soul who did her best but appealed to the lowest common denominator of her charges – this was guaranteed to irritate Keith. I asked the Social Worker if he could go to somewhere a bit more stimulating. She managed to arrange for him to go to a place the other side of Norwich. This was in a purpose-built building and associated with the Hellesdon Mental Hospital. I hoped the staff there would have a better understanding of his needs and that he would settle there. Again I had to take him and probably I should have been prepared to stay until he got used to it but I was a bit desperate by then and was glad when they offered to bring him home at the end of the session. He attacked what appeared to him to be two strange women when they tried to get him to get into a strange car, and on another occasion he even attacked his own daughter when she tried to save me a journey by taking him on the way to her work, in her (strange) car. The Respite Centre refused to have him any more.

CHAPTER 3

Disadvantages of ignorance and isolation

I then asked the Social Worker to get me some help in the house. I had had a retired Home Help who came to tidy the house for one and a half hours a week but she became ill and when she recovered her transport broke down and I felt it was time she retired properly.

The Social Services used an Agency who seemed to have no idea of what was needed. The first person they sent me was a retired army man who had recently been a driving examiner. As you may imagine, he did not get on well with Keith and did not last long. The next 'help' was a single mother who, understandably, felt her children needed her more than the money - she only came once. Our daughter, using another agency, found me Michael. He had no training but had experience with his father. He did no work for me in the house but was a good companion for Keith. He lived in Norwich and had no car. The bus passed his door but the only one that came to this village took about an hour because it came via all the little villages. Michael arrived at about 10 am and had to leave at 2.30 pm. I had to pay for the bus both ways and pay Michael for the two hours he spent on the bus. I could only go out without Keith if Michael took him to lunch at the Pub - for which I had to pay of course. We could, no doubt, have worked out a modus vivendi but at this point I broke down. I could see and hear what Keith wanted but could not say anything or move. I probably went to sleep or fainted as the next thing I knew was opening my eyes to find I was alone and the phone was ringing. I struggled to my feet and found the call was from our 92 year old neighbour who Keith had asked to call the doctor for me. I assured her I was OK now

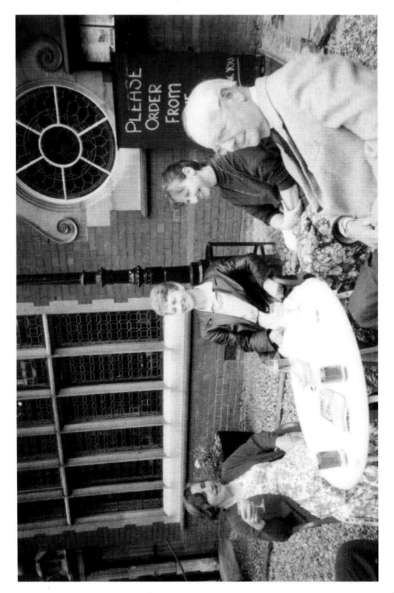

With all three daughters on the same continent for once.

and as I was very cold I crawled into bed. I was awakened by a man I did not know asking 'What happened?' He was the doctor on emergency duty. He took my pulse and asked me a lot of questions, then he left telling me I would be better when I had had a good rest – what a hope! When Keith could not so much as make a cup of tea.

After a few days we received a notification that a bed was available at Dr Tawse's specially designed and built hospital connected with the West Norwich Hospital where Keith had been to have his eyes tested. Michael came to be with Keith while I drove our own car. Unfortunately Keith refused to stay and Dr Tawse would not see him or use any means to get him to stay without the sanction of the Mental Health Act. We waited three hours in the hope that Keith would change his mind, but he would not so we drove home again. The next step was to get him 'sectioned' under the Mental Health Act which took away power from the patient and his family and gave it to the medical experts. I was distressed at having to do this but feared that I might die before he did and it was better for him to be cared for by younger people, giving me some respite and hopefully I would then be able to soften the blow by visiting him frequently.

After six weeks in hospital, I was told that he must spend the rest of his life in a secure EMI (Elderly Mentally Infirm) Residential Home and I was given a list to choose from. I don't know what I expected but it was a great shock to think he would never come home again. Very little was said at the hospital about how Keith was assessed although I visited every other day. When I was away for a few days with my sister in Kent, our eldest granddaughter (30 years old and living in Ipswich) visited Keith and was very upset because he told her there had been a terrible mistake and he should not be in hospital at all. She came with me another time and agreed that while he looked the same, sometimes he was rational and sometimes not. He seemed to come and go. He continued to be able to shave himself with an electric shaver I had bought him and I managed to cut his hair so he looked normal, but although he was physically fit, his brain was no longer reliable.

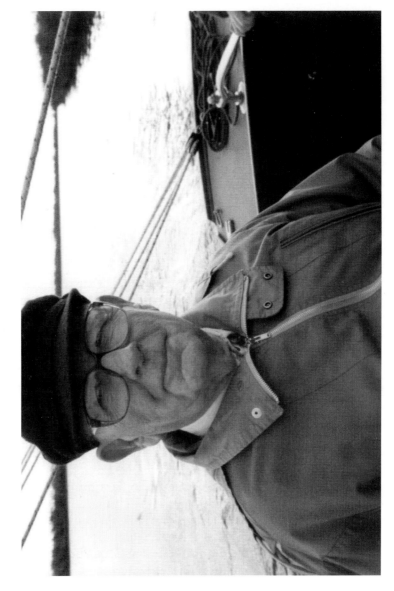

After he became blind he still loved sailing, but there had to be another hand on the tiller.

CHAPTER 4

Even the best Residential Homes are not perfect

I had no idea what to look for in choosing a Residential Home. I had known Keith for 60 years but he was a very different person now. He had been a lifelong Socialist but had trained as an architect and appreciated good design and classical music. He was a Planning Inspector before he retired and held Public Local Enquiries where he was treated with great respect and had to hold himself aloof so that he did not appear to be taking sides. He was always interested in ethics and philosophy but not 'churchianity'. He loved children and young people and worked (voluntarily) for Quakers as Registering Officer for Marriages and he mixed equally happily with admirals, bishops and builders' labourers.

I managed to make a short list of five Residential Homes, and our youngest daughter (the other children were in New Zealand, Africa or London) took me in her Land Rover to see them one afternoon. We agreed on one that was near enough for frequent visits, not too large as to be impersonal but large enough to have a choice of companions and to justify equipment. The owner and manager was a State Registered Nurse, and she and her family lived on the premises. She had had a lot of experience and liked looking after EMI people. Being a trained nurse we expected and found she had a good relationship with the doctor. This was important to us as Keith had already had one change of doctor and appointments were not easy to get. We did not want him to suffer any lack of medical attention if it should be needed. This building was roomy and attractive and had a lively outlook over the village green. We were also encouraged to visit and take him out whenever we liked. There was a garden and two cats. None of the residents took any

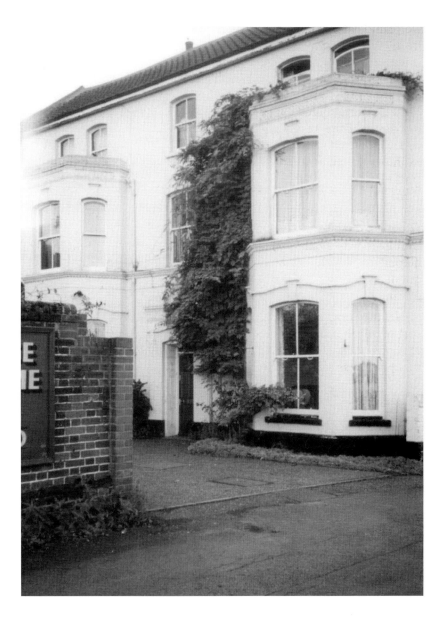

The Home we chose for him.

notice of these but we thought they added to the homely atmosphere. Of course nothing in this life is perfect. On the down side we found later nearly all the staff were untrained girls and boys from the village, spectacles and hearing aids got mixed up and as it was almost impossible to sort them out they were never worn. The residents had a nice bedroom each and were encouraged to have their own things around them but as one of the residents helped herself to other peoples' things the rooms were kept locked during the day, but the key was always given to me whenever I asked for it. I was never given a satisfactory reason as to why none of the rooms, even the toilets, had any means of identification. The night staff were expected to get everybody up and ready for breakfast by 7 am so there was little time to be patient with people who did not feel co-operative at that time in the morning, or had strong views about what they would wear. They were therefore bundled into whatever was available and easiest to get on. Incontinence, not helped by the difficulty of finding the lavatory, necessitated frequent laundering of clothes which sometimes were not available on time or no longer fitted.

In the mornings I believe there were visiting therapists of one sort or another but I always visited in the afternoons and found the inmates rather bored and sometimes fights broke out. The cost of this place was £218 per week, which was cheap as these places go. The Social Services would have paid this after I had used up most of our savings, and would have left me the house. However as I now have less than half my husband's income and none of his tax allowances I am glad of the interest on our savings as well as preferring to be independent. Although he never complained, I know Keith was not happy, and I was distressed that I had not felt able to keep him at home or perhaps had chosen the wrong Home for him.

CHAPTER 5

He did not know me and I was very confused about our relationship

During the Spring and Summer months I visited Keith twice a week and often took him out to places he used to enjoy. He never knew who I was or recognised any of the places I took him to, but he thanked me for being kind enough to visit him and thought it was wonderful that I knew about things and places that he used to know very well. My neighbours also visited him twice. He said 'I do not know who you are but I feel very honoured that you have come to see me.' When they visited the second time they gave him a banana which he ate with great enthusiasm. I thereafter took bananas as I thought they were probably better for him than the chocolate bars which I had been taking for him, and certainly not so messy. Once when he had deteriorated quite a bit, he ate the skin as well and pronounced it 'disgusting'! From then on I took tissues to wipe our hands and mouths and removed the skin before I gave a banana to him. He was very pleased to have the tissues to mop himself up after he had eaten. He also enjoyed tapes of classical music that I took with a portable player. He could not manage the player by himself and the tapes disappeared if I left them. He could, however, tell if the tape finished before the music reached its finale.

He did not always seem to notice when I visited even when I had a friend with me he used to know well, but when I said 'We must go now' he always jumped up and said 'Oh no! don't go!'

I knew our daughter would visit her father whenever she could so when the winter came and I was afraid I would become clinically depressed living alone in the isolated house, I arranged to go to Birmingham to the Centre for Quaker Studies called

16

Woodbrooke. They had a part-time course in association with Birmingham University Theology Department. I would spend two terms studying there and two years writing up at home. This seemed to be just what I wanted as I have always enjoyed studying, and not having to think about meals or anything else was just the break I needed. The course consisted of two essays of 4,000 words on taught material and a dissertation on a religious aspect of your choice, leading to a Masters degree. I proposed to use the spiritual aspects of dementia for my dissertation. To my delight and amazement I found there had been a conference at Woodbrooke on dementia and I met people who had been inspired by Tom Kitwood (see Chapter 6). His colleague was a Quaker and had asked for this Conference of which I was shown the file. I also met several people who played various roles at The Retreat (which had been opened in 1796 and was still treating the whole person whatever their mental problems) and social workers who had met people with dementia in their work and felt their problems were not properly understood. They were as anxious as I was that the remaining part of the person whose brain had been attacked by dementia should be responded to as any other human being, and not cut off from society by unreasonable fear and unthinking distaste and a lack of understanding of what makes us human. I was given many contacts and felt I had to follow them up there and then whatever my supervisor thought about it. My Master's degree went out of the window but the many who had suffered, or had recognised lack of appreciation of spirituality or personhood in others, made this book a necessary priority.

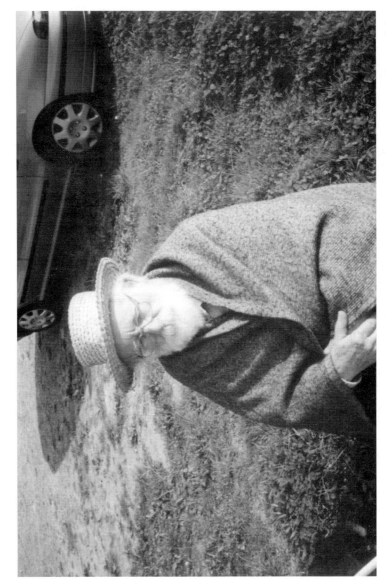

Last picture of him, by the river but not aware of it. Wearing my hat because the sun was too hot and the picnic blanket because he was too cold.

CHAPTER 6

Alzheimer and Kitwood

Doctors and social workers have to deal with a wide variety of social and medical ills so it is not surprising that they find it difficult to keep up with all that has recently been discovered. Dementia has been with us since earliest times and has been explained in various ways. At one time all suffering was seen as punishment for the sins of the sufferer or predecessors, and mental problems were explained as possession by an evil spirit of some sort; later on humans were assumed to have reverted to being animals, and a more recent idea was that the spirit goes and leaves the (still living) body behind. None of these explanations was believed by everybody all the time but they have left behind attitudes that, lacking any firm facts, have coloured the way diseases of the brain have been ignored or misunderstood for too long.

Dr Alois Alzheimer made his discovery in 1906 but it was not until the 1960s that Brain Science was taken seriously. Tom Kitwood complained that even then there were not available non-invasive methods of measuring the neuro-chemical effects of otherwise simple treatments. He also pointed to the good effect on confused elderly people of Reality Orientation, which was originally developed in the 1950s for men traumatized by war.

Tom Kitwood came to the study of dementia in an unusual way but gave unstintingly of his exceptional insights and creativity. His first degree was from Cambridge where he specialised in bio-chemistry. He worked for some time in Uganda and in Britain as a school teacher and chaplain and at the same time co-authored a textbook on organic-chemistry. He was awarded an MSc in Psychology and Sociology of Education and later a PhD in Social Psychology from Bradford University. While at Bradford his wife brought home an

19

elderly lady she had been helping to choose a pain-killer in a super-market. They became friendly with this old lady and were horri-fied to find she had been put in a huge depressing and isolated Residential Home where she soon died.

Tom Kitwood felt ashamed that with all his learning he had been taken in by the Standard Paradigm that she had suffered 'the death that leaves the body behind'. I felt the same, without his learn-ing but having known and lived closely for many years with the person who looked the same but seemed somehow lost. Bob Woods, Professor of Clinical Psychology of the Elderly at the University of Wales at Bangor, in his speech at Bradford celebrating the life and work of Tom Kitwood, who died in November 1998 at the early age of 61, said that he had to admit that he had accepted the Standard Paradigm and that it was widely held by many people.

Tom Kitwood had only started working on dementia ten years ago when he was asked by two psychiatrists and a clinical psy-chologist to give them academic support and research supervision in their work on dementia. As a result of this he found, when exam-ining the brain of a deceased dementia sufferer, that although the plaques and tangles that Alzheimer found were undoubtedly there, they did not seem to him to cause sufficient damage to explain the degree of deterioration that the patient had suffered. He invented the term Malignant Social Psychology to explain what so often hap-pens and he developed a means of measuring this so that it could be avoided. He called this Dementia Care Mapping (DCM). I here give a list of headings that Tom Kitwood used to demonstrate how personhood of someone with dementia was often undermined:

1. TREACHERY - using forms of deception in order to distract or manipulate a person or force them into compliance.

2. DISEMPOWERMENT - not allowing a person to use the abil-ities they do have; failing to help them to complete actions that they have initiated.

3. INFANTILIZATION - treating a person very patronizingly, as an insensitive parent might treat a very young child.

4. INTIMIDATION - inducing fear in a person through the use of threats or physical power.

5. LABELLING - using a category such as Dementia, as the main basis for interacting with a person and for explaining their behaviour.

6. STIGMATIZATION - treating a person as if they were a diseased object, an alien or an outcast.

7. OUTPACING - providing information, presenting choices etc., at a rate too fast for a person to understand; putting them under pressure to do things more rapidly than they can bear.

8. INVALIDATION - failing to acknowledge the subjective reality of a person's experience, especially what they are feeling.

9. BANISHMENT - sending a person away or excluding them - physically or psychologically.

10. OBJECTIFICATION - treating a person as if they were a lump of dead matter: to be pushed, lifted, filled, pumped or drained without proper reference to the fact that they are sentient beings.

These questions, and others that were added later, were used for training and assessment in Residential Homes and Tom Kitwood was invited to America to explain and demonstrate their use. He and his DCM were very well received there.

Tom Kitwood noted that the service to mental health in this country was seriously underfunded and advised that a career structure was vital to attract the calibre of staff needed to raise the standards in what had been a Cinderella service. He also noted that ideas such as his had been held by others from time to time but had somehow been ignored. He himself appears to have ignored the difficulties of lone elderly carers in rural situations and the difficulties in the case of small homes where the requirements of hygiene and the Health and Safety Act as well as finance, make the running and maintenance particularly burdensome.

CHAPTER 7

Churches' attitudes, training and law

I had hoped that the Churches Together in England might develop a joint view about dementia instead of spending so much time and energy on creedal differences. (Keith had always had strong feelings against getting involved in creedal disagreements.) The Methodists, under Rev. Albert Jewell, have appreciated that there was a need in their Homes for old people, but have concentrated on reviving memories of past beliefs. Some people have recognisable spirituality without having ever belonged to any organised religion. The Churches Together in Newcastle have worked together with others who are interested in this problem and although calling themselves a Christian Council, their Working Group on Dementia seems to appreciate that some form of spirituality is an integral part of universal humanity.

The Theological Department of Birmingham University suggested I should read Stephen Pattison's three books on the subject. After much difficulty I did obtain them and found that he had, at different times, been the official chaplain at several mental institutions. He had not felt that his training at Theological College had prepared him adequately for this work and he was appalled at the lack of money, attention and skilled treatment that the people he tried to serve, received.

As early as 1714, Thomas Story, speaking of the old age of William Penn (Quaker Faith and Practice 21.62), said 'His memory was almost quite lost, and the use of his understanding suspended, so that he was not so conversible as formerly; and yet as near the Truth, in the love of it, as before. His mind was in an innocent state, as appeared by his very loving deportment to all that came near him: and that he still had a good sense of Truth was plain, by some very clear sentences he spoke in the Life and Power of truth in an evening meeting we had together there; wherein we were greatly comforted; so that I was ready to think this was a sort of sequestration of him from all the concerns of this life which so much oppressed him, not in judgement but in mercy, that he might have rest, and not be oppressed thereby to the end.'

In 1792 William Tuke, a Quaker tea merchant in York, England, and (independently) Philippe Pinel, an agnostic medical man in charge of institutions for the mentally ill in Paris, France, both felt that the mentally ill were human and should not be treated as if they had no feelings. Pinel removed the shackles and other degrading forms of restraint and Tuke proceeded to build a beautiful building on a healthy site, where it still stands today, and used what was then called 'Moral Treatment'. This 'moral treatment' was very popular for a time but the huge asylums, as they were then called, did not lend themselves to moral treatment and they became little better than warehouses and they and their unfortunate inmates got a bad name. Eventually it was thought that Care in the Community was better for everyone and so the problem has arrived at my door and possibly yours too, regardless of lack of training and in some areas, little or no support.

I have already mentioned Wordsworth and Tom Kitwood mentions doctors and carers who speak as if they believe the Standard Paradigm but act quite differently. Tom Kitwood himself said he felt quite guilty going against the (apparently) general belief. Thank goodness he did, and hopefully he will not be forgotten.

At one time those certified as mentally inadequate for any reason were deliberately denied a vote. Now they have a vote in theory but it is almost impossible for them to use it. When my husband was registered blind and living at home, he was on the electoral role and I was permitted to go into the voting booth to help him make his mark in the appropriate place. When he was in the Residential Home he was on their electoral role but there was no one responsible to see he was able to use his right to vote. I had continuing Power of Attorney over his financial affairs, though he signed papers when he was still able to know what he was doing. Could some similar arrangement be made for a Proxy vote? This is a very important Human Right, and so long as it appears to be denied them they will appear to be less than human and nobody will notice if they tend to be treated less than humanely.

My husband died on 6th March 2001. We had celebrated our Golden Wedding in 1991 and he was diagnosed as having macular degeneration in 1993.

It is difficult to say exactly when the blindness or the dementia started. Looking back, the inappropriate changing of lanes on the Norwich outer ring road and the injury to a dog soon afterwards in South Walsham by an otherwise experienced and careful driver, were both probably caused by minor strokes. Before we were sent to the eye hospital Keith described all masts and tall poles as being crooked and appearing to have bites taken out of them.

I suppose I should have suspected dementia when he caught the next train home and offered no explanation, and when plays and concerts no longer held any interest for him. His blindness was not total - he had peripheral vision, and determination to remain in charge and not talk about what he considered mundane matters - all this was part of his character. He often complained about his memory but it did not seem to me to be worse than mine or that of anybody else of his age. However, when he did not recognise any of his family and friends or any of the places he used to know so well, the alarm bells could not be ignored any longer.

He was in his own home for six years and although we tried several ways to ease the domestic situation we never once talked about the possibility that he might have to go into a Residential Home. I don't think he would have ever accepted that this was a possible necessity unless he had met the idea before it could possibly relate to him. That is the main reason why I have written this. The general public has not expected to live so long or to have to take responsibility for one another, particularly when minds fail while the body still seems nearly as fit and strong as ever. We all need to know that this can happen, just as we have learned to accept that death and bereavement, cancer and other ills are all part of normal life with which adults often have to cope. It is saddest when it happens to the young, but even then it is better not to let ignorance and emotion get in the way of friendly contact and sharing of time and feeling.

Being human and alive is wonderful. Don't take it for granted.

Keith could have had an X-ray and possibly an operation to prolong his life a little, but it would have been very frightening for him, and possibly for the hospital staff too. There seemed no hope of a cure for his dementia and as he was already 84 it seemed kinder to let him slip away naturally where he had lived for two years and with his wife and daughter with him, even if he did not know them - at least they were not in strange uniforms.

By the way, Alzheimer's is used as a general name for various sorts of dementia. Different causes of dementia behave slightly differently and of course different people respond differently, so this is more of a general warning and not detailed information.

When you feel that not only does no one understand but you get the feeling (rightly or wrongly) that friends and relations and even one's own church do not want to understand or even know about what you are both experiencing it makes for a very rough and weary road to follow. You have no previous experience to fall back on and no light at the end of the tunnel.

Our daughter and I were told that the night before he died Keith said 'Dear darling Margaret, are you enjoying your supper?' This was how he used to speak to me when he was feeling affectionate. The fact that it was addressed to a pink plush covered armchair did not prevent the lump in my throat.

I hope you will not have the experience that my husband and I had to grapple with, but if you do you will know you are not alone and perhaps this book will help you, and others, avoid some of the pitfalls and the mistakes that we made.

If you have read this with compassionate understanding you will have set me free to enjoy what is left of my life in peace.

Thank you.

Bibliography

Books, Papers and Journals I have read during
this experience

Allan, Kate, *Communication and Consultation Exploring ways for staff to involve people with dementia in developing services (the comprehensive dementia reference book for the year 2000)*, Joseph Rowntree Foundation, 2001.

Alzheimer's Society magazine and other publications.

Bayley, John, *Iris - A memoir of Iris Murdoch* Abacus, 1999.

Barrance, Sue, *Dementia Voice – Blackberry Hill Hospital*, unpublished research.

Bonhoeffer, Dietrich, *Letters and Papers from Prison (an abridged edition)*, SCM Classics, SCM Press, 2001.

Cayton, Harry, Dr Nori Graham, Dr James Warner, *Alzheimers at Your Fingertips*, Class Publishing, London, 1997.

Cherry, Charles, *A Quiet Haven*, Fairleigh Dickinson University Press, Rutherford, New Jersey, 1989.

Civil Service magazine

Coleman, Professor Peter, unpublished chapter for Open University.

Digby, Ann, *Madness Morality and Medicine*, Cambridge University Press, 1985.

Fletcher, Rev. Joseph, *Indicators of Humanhood*, quoted by Hugo Petzsch.

Foskett, Canon John, *Meaning in Madness*, Tiptree, England, 1984.

Foster, Margaret, *Have the Men had Enough?*, Chatto and Windus Ltd, London, 1989.

Goldsmith, Malcolm, *Hearing the Voice of People with Dementia,* Jessica Kingsley, 1996.

Grant, Linda, *Remind me Who I am Again,* Granta Books, GB, 1998.

Greenfield, Professor Susan, *The Brain Story,* Oxford University Press.

Jewell, Rev. Albert, Editor *Spirituality and Ageing,* Jessica Kingsley, 1998.

Kitwood, Tom, *Dementia Reconsidered,* Open University Press, 1997.

Newsletter of the Dementia Working Party Newcastle

Pattison, Stephen, *Pastoral Care and Liberation Theology,* SPCK, 1997.

Petzsch, Hugo, *A Study of Attitudes to Dementing People,* Occasional paper for Edinburgh University.

Quaker Faith and Practice: the book of Christian discipline of the Yearly Meeting of the Religious Society of Friends, The Yearly Meeting of the Religious Society of Friends (Quakers) in Britain, 1995.

Sacks, Oliver, *The man who mistook his wife for a hat,* Pan Books, 1986.

Sansom, Carolyn, Ph D thesis for University of Wales.

Stewart, Kathleen Anne, *The York Retreat in the light of the Quaker Way,* William Sessions Limited, York, England, 1992.

Teilhard de Chardin, Pierre, *The Phenomenon of Man,* Fontana Books, 1965.

The Journal of Dementia Care Vol. 7 No. 1, *Tributes to Tom Kitwood,* Jan/Feb 1999.

Tibbs, Margaret Ann, Paper for Alzheimer's Society.

Treetops, Rev. Jackie, *A Daisy among the Dandelions,* Faith in Elderly People project, Leeds, May 1991.

Various Quaker publications.

Wells, H.G., *Outline of History,* Cassell & Co. Ltd, 1920.

Woods, Professor Bob, *Caring for the Person with Dementia (a guide for families and other carers),* 1996.

USEFUL CONTACT

Alzheimer's Society
Gordon House
10 Greencoat Place
London SW1P 1PH

Tel 020 7306 0606
Email enquiries@alzheimers.org.uk